MEDICAL ZEN

MEDICAL ZEN

Fit in 15

A scientifically designed fifteen-minute daily wellness exercise program that will dramatically improve your metabolic rate and overall level of fitness so you can

rip through *calories*,
have more *energy*,
improve your *health*,

and *accelerate* your *weight loss*.

Michael R. Keller, MD

Copyright © 2009 by Michael R. Keller, MD.

Library of Congress Control Number: 2009908456
ISBN: Hardcover   978-1-4415-6552-5
             Softcover   978-1-4415-6551-8

All rights reserved. No part of this book may be reproduced or transmitted in any form or by any means, electronic or mechanical, including photocopying, recording, or by any information storage and retrieval system, without permission in writing from the copyright owner.

This book was printed in the United States of America.

To order additional copies of this book, contact:
Xlibris Corporation
1-888-795-4274
www.Xlibris.com
Orders@Xlibris.com
67428

Dedicated to all of the patients I had the privilege to meet, help, and learn from, thank you all

Obesity is the number one health care crisis in America today!

MEDICAL ZEN
Fit in 15

A scientifically designed fifteen-minute daily wellness exercise program done in the morning right after waking up that will dramatically improve your metabolic rate so you can rip through calories, have more energy, improve your health, and accelerate your weight loss.

The most optimal time to exercise is in the morning. Why? Because you will get more out of it throughout the day than you will by exercising in the afternoon or night. If you are a NASCAR driver and you are about to start a race, do you just turn on your car and go? No, you will lose badly, and all the nice endorsements will *poof!* vanish. What they do is warm up their car. Why? Because they know a warm engine performs much more efficiently. Peak performance occurs when the engine is *warm*. You are no different. You are a machine. By warming up your machine in the morning, a lot of *magic* will occur. You will double the amount of calories you burn, you will burn sugar more efficiently, you will have more energy, you will be in a better mood, you will delay the aging process, you will lose much more weight . . . and more.

Unfortunately, the favorite way for Americans to wake up in the morning is with a cup of coffee, a cigarette, or a Mountain Dew.

Medical Zen: Fit in 15 is much more than just a weight loss program. It is a complete fitness routine that will bring balance to your life and improve your health and overall levels of fitness.

You will see significant improvement in the following:

Metabolic rate and sugar metabolism (ability to burn calories)
Energy
Flexibility
Core strength and stamina
Balance and coordination
Focus, concentration, and memory
Joint pain and stiffness
Bone density
Cardiovascular performance (including improvements in blood pressure and heart rate)

And finally . . . *accelerated weight loss!*

I am a family practice physician, and I have been studying my patients for over twenty years, learning and passing along the behaviors, dietary habits, and exercise philosophies that repeatedly work in improving their overall health. I have also been studying the miraculous benefits of Eastern medical philosophies for the past four years and have designed a fifteen-minute program that targets all aspects of fitness and blends Western medical concerns and approaches with *time-tested* Eastern exercise and breathing techniques.

The result:

A complete exercise program that encompasses all aspects of health and fitness

Flexibility
Overall joint mobility: Arthritis is the number one contributing cause of disability in adults, and poor flexibility is the leading contributor to premature joint aging and arthritis.

Cardiovascular Performance
The ability to pump and circulate blood efficiently: Heart attacks are still the number one cause of death for men and women over age fifty. Millions of people suffer from high blood pressure, requiring them to take medications daily to control it.

Core Muscle Strength and Stamina
Core muscle power and how long it can be used: Injury relates more to a failure in muscle stamina rather than in muscle strength. Muscles are the second most active body part that consumes oxygen. (What is the first? It's the *brain*.)

Breathing
The ability to oxygenate the blood and provide energy to the body: Most Americans breathe very inefficiently and actually waste energy breathing. Asthma is the most common physically limiting disease in children. Millions of Americans suffer with asthma as adults.

Balance and Coordination
Falling is a huge risk at any age but more so as you get older: Hip and pelvic fractures are frequently fatal because of the secondary blood clots

they cause. Balance and coordination are *learned* processes that you reteach yourself every day. You forget what you do not practice.

Bone Health
Osteoporosis affects one in two women over the age of seventy: Bone density begins to erode for most women after age forty. Women that suffer from a hip or pelvic fracture have a 25 percent chance (that's one in four) to die due to secondary complications that relate to blood clots. Osteoporosis is becoming much more common now in men.

Visualization
Mental focus exercises the mind: Alzheimer's is a scary reality for many elderly people. The brain is the greediest organ when it comes to using and burning oxygen. The brain requires daily stimulation to keep it active and healthy.

Keep in mind that success starts with *believing in yourself.*

Most exercise programs do not touch on all aspects of fitness. A few popular exercise routines like P90X and thai bo that get great "physical results" focus on strength, stamina, and flexibility. But in my opinion, they do not highlight or instruct on the benefits of medical breathing, the reduction of inflammatory factors, the improvement in bone density, and do not promote visualization to improve mental stimulation.

Most exercise routines are lacking in some way. This program targets all aspects of fitness and the added benefit is . . . you also *maximize weight loss.*

Eastern medical philosophies have packaged the earth into five key energies. Five thousand years ago, advanced scientific tools, other than keen observation, were absent; so the monks and scholars used generic labeling to better understand, document, and pass down the knowledge of their discoveries on how our bodies, the world, and the universe operated.

Those five key energies are called the five elements, and the science behind them is called the

Five Elemental Theory
Wood—Fire—Earth—Metal—Water

What are some of the energies they reflect? How about mechanical like joint mobility, or hydraulic like pressure in the arteries or viscosity of blood, or biochemical such as the consumption of oxygen to produce energy, or bioelectric along a nerve fiber, and yes, even quantum mechanics—all outlined in the East going back five thousand years. We are just not familiar with their terminology, so we assume that we in the West figured it out first. We did not.

I have taken what I have learned and blended a program to fit Western expectations and time constraints. We all have at least fifteen minutes to be healthy . . . no excuses!

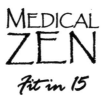

The program laid out has nine key exercises that should be done as soon as you wake up every morning, six days a week. This is the commitment to *you*. Every day you exercise, you get younger; and every day you don't, you get much older. To stay healthy and lose weight and to keep it off, you need to increase your metabolic rate on a daily basis. The best time to do this is in the morning. You need to warm up your engine so it performs better throughout the day, and like a nice warm car, it takes time to cool down. You can double your calorie burn throughout the day by exercising in the morning.

The exercises are broken down from beginner to intermediate to advanced. It will take a while to get used to the exercises, but the beginning program should be accomplished in about five minutes, intermediate in ten, and advanced in fifteen.

The *key* is to do the exercises *continuously without rest.*

Focus!

Start with the following schedule:

Week 1: Get familiar with the program—Monday through Saturday morning

Week 2-4: Beginner five-minute program—Monday through Saturday morning

Week 5-8: Intermediate ten-minute program—Monday through Saturday morning

Week 8-12: Advanced fifteen-minute program—Monday through Saturday morning

Week 12 onward: Continue the morning routine. Never give it up and don't let anyone take it away from you.

Being healthy is your gift to yourself.

Keep in mind you only get in what you get out. If you are lazy, you will get nothing. If you push yourself, you should expect, on average, about fifteen pounds weight loss in three months. Don't worry if you are already thin, you will not lose weight unless you need to. Remember the key is *balanced health and fitness for the rest of your life!*

Never stop and keep pushing yourself!

The Program

Metal Element:

Improving Breathing and Oxygenation

It Starts with Breathing

Westerners are taught to breathe from the chest. This type of breathing is very inefficient. The majority of the blood that circulates through the lungs is located in the lower or bottom third. Chest breathing focuses the air in the mid to upper lung regions that are not as rich with blood as the lower third. If you have ever watched an infant, they breathe from the lower abdomen—abdominal breathing—because they innately know that this is the most efficient way to breathe. A key to increasing your own metabolic rate is to get as much energy-rich oxygen into the lower lung so that it can superoxygenate the blood. This requires abdominal breathing. Also, keep in mind that breathing is the primary way the body excretes or eliminates waste. By improving your breathing, not only are you supercharging your cells with more oxygen, you are also cleaning your body by eliminating more waste!

The type of breathing that this program follows is called *fire path breathing* because it helps supercharge your internal energy and makes it flow.

1. Breathe in through the nose.
2. Breathe out through the nose.
3. As you breathe in, press tongue against the roof of your mouth.
4. As you breathe out, drop tongue to the floor of the mouth.
5. Breathe in. Push the air to the lower abdomen.
6. Breathe out. Pull your belly button to your spine.
7. Pull up the anal area called the *hui yin*. At the same time, closing and lifting the anal area prevents energy leakage.

8. As you breathe in, follow the energy up the spine and over the head to a point on the forehead between the eyebrows, lighting that point up (visualization).
9. Breathe out and let the energy drop to the lower abdomen, stoking the fire (visualization).

Try this breathing technique standing up about ten times right now.

Apply fire path breathing to all exercises.

The Importance of Visualization

You *are* what you *think*. This is an oversimplification, but I can divide my patients immediately on who *will succeed* and who *will not* by their mental outlook. *If* you can see yourself successful, you will succeed; and if you hem and haw and whine and moan about what you need to do, then you will fail. It *is* as simple as that. Visualization is an important key in the success of this program. It is the cornerstone of the mental stimulation that exercises the brain and keeps the brain healthy and young. The other aspect is maximizing the delivery of energy, oxygen, and nutrition.

Exercise No. 1 Embrace the Heart

- Head up
- Shoulders relaxed, down
- Chest hollow and kidneys pushed back
- Tailbone tucked in
- Feet shoulder width apart with knees slightly bent
- Arms at heart level, rounded out in front of you like you're holding a large beach ball with the palms facing toward your chest

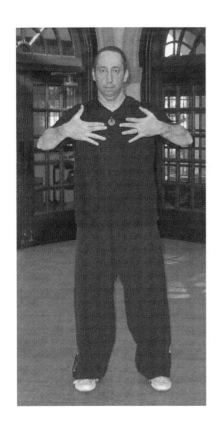
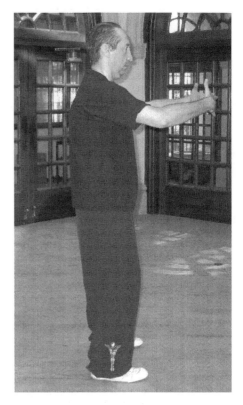

Breathe in though the nose (fire path breathing, see above) with your tongue on the roof of your mouth, up the back of the spine, lighting up your sixth chakra (the point between your eyebrows); then exhale down the front to the lower abdominal area, stoking the fire in the lower abdomen, what is called the brass basin. The brass basin is the lower internal abdominal and pelvic area that acts like an energy reservoir. As you breathe, you *deposit* energy into it; and with each breath, you stoke the energy or fire, making it bigger and bigger, charging up the battery to help you through your day (remember visualization).

Breathing cycle is two seconds in and two seconds out.

Beginner: Start with five breath cycles
Intermediate: Ten breath cycles
Advanced: Fifteen breath cycles

Key points in the exercise

- Stay relaxed.
- Breathe deep into the lower abdomen and relax the chest and shoulders.
- Visualize. As you breathe in, you are bringing the oxygen and energy up the spine to your brain, lighting up at the point between your eyebrows like a beacon (sixth chakra). This provides needed oxygen and nutrition to the brain.
- Then as you breathe out, drop that energy down the front and deposit it into the lower abdominal area, increasing the energy with each breath. This is called stoking the fire.
- Visualization is key, and this starts the process of increasing your metabolic rate.

Physical and Physiological Benefits

1. Increases cellular metabolic rate for maximal calorie burn
2. Superoxygenates the blood, providing the critical energetic fuel that feeds the cells
3. Strengthens the diaphragm, which improves breathing efficiency, which allows for improved oxygen and carbon dioxide transfer—more of the good in and more of the bad out
4. Massages the internal organs, stimulating and energizing them
5. Dramatically increases the oxygen and energy delivered to the brain
6. Stimulates the brain activity
7. Activates the second heart (the abdomen), improving blood flow and cardiovascular performance
8. Charges the abdomen battery, which is energy to be used later in the day
9. Initiates the release of endorphins that reduce pain and improve mood

Potential Medical Health Benefits

1. Blood pressure reduction
2. Resting heart rate reduction
3. Improved asthma
4. Improved bowel function: constipation
5. Improved energy: chronic fatigue
6. Improved mood: depression and anxiety
7. Improved focus and attention
8. Improved memory
9. Reduced pain

Exercise No. 2 Gather the Sun and Press the Earth

Starting position

- Head up
- Shoulders relaxed, down
- Chest hollow and kidneys pushed back
- Tailbone tucked in,
- Feet shoulder width apart with knees slightly bent
- Arms out to your sides, arms crossed in front of you at waist level

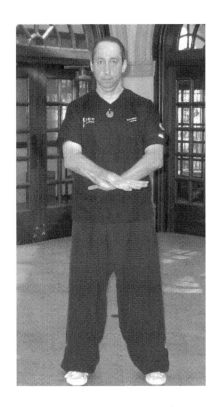

As You Are Breathing In (Fire Path Breathing):

Lift your crossed arms over your head and then swing them down off to each side and back around in front of your chest, gathering the energy.

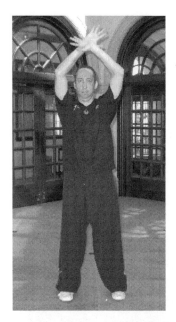
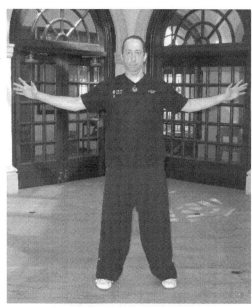
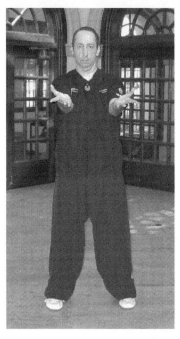
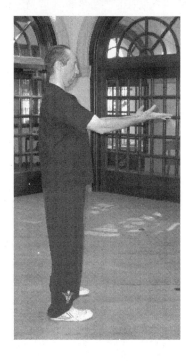

Then pull your arms and the energy they hold toward you, rubbing your sides, and then push the energy into your kidneys (midback) with your hands and arch your back. This is one continuous motion.

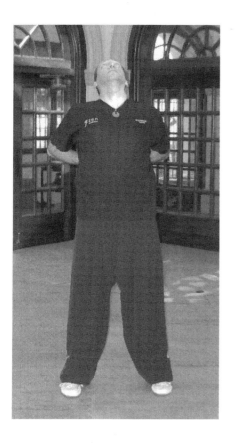
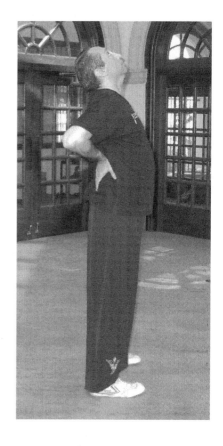

As You Breathe Out (Fire Path Breathing):

Rub your hands down your back over your buttocks, down the back of your legs, while bending at the waist, and then swing your arms forward once they reach the ankles and touch the ground.

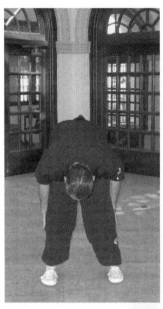

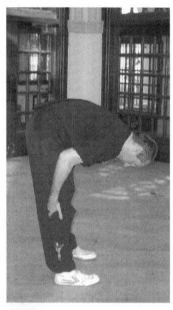

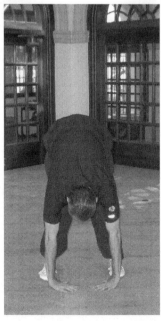

Breathe In (Fire Path Breathing):

Rub your hands up the inside of both legs and over the groin area. As you rise up, lift hands and arms to shoulder height. Hands should be pointed toward each other, palms facing down.

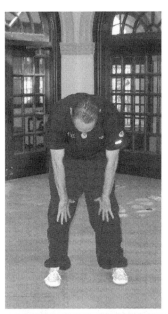
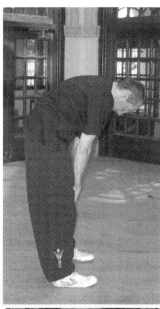
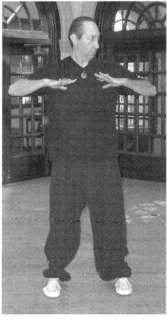
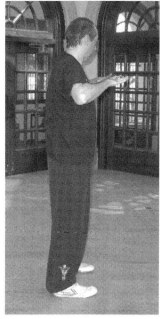

Breathe Out (Fire Path Breathing):
Push the palms down and look left.

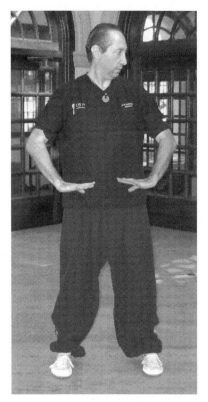
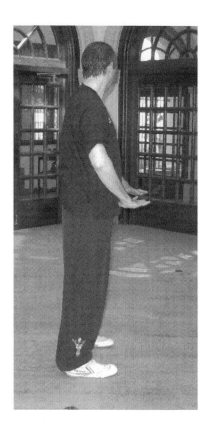

This is one complete exercise cycle.

Beginner: Three exercise cycles
Intermediate: Six cycles
Advanced: Nine cycles

Each breathing cycle (breathing in then out) is three seconds in and three seconds out.

Key Points

- Visualize gathering the energy with your arms and then pushing it into your kidney area.

- Rubbing is actually massaging energy meridians that help move energy in your body.
- When bending at the waist, just bend to the degree that feels comfortable; you do not have to touch the floor.

Physical and Physiological Benefits

1. Further increases cellular metabolic rate
2. Continues to superoxygenate the blood
3. Further strengthens the diaphragm, improving breathing efficiency, which allows for improved oxygen and carbon dioxide transfer
4. Massages the internal organs more directly, further stimulating and energizing them
5. Maximizes the oxygen and energy delivered to the brain
6. Continues the stimulation of the brain and brain activity
7. Improves the second heart's (the abdomen) ability to improve blood flow
8. Further charges the abdomen battery, which is energy to be used later in the day
9. Continues the release of endorphins that reduce pain and improve mood
10. Improves spinal flexibility
11. Activates the energy meridians to improve energy throughout the body

Potential Medical Health Benefits

1. Blood pressure
2. Resting heart rate
3. Asthma
4. Bowel function: constipation
5. Energy: chronic fatigue

6. Mood: depression and anxiety
7. Focus and attention
8. Memory
9. Lower and midback arthritis
10. Lower and midback chronic pain
11. Neck pain and arthritis
12. Chronic pain in general

Wood Element:

Improving Flexibility and Releasing Stress

Exercise No. 3 Midline Stretch

- Position feet shoulder width apart.
- Point toes forward.
- Lock knees back.
- Tuck chin to chest.
- Place hands behind head or neck and let the arms fold forward across the face.
- Bend down slowly at the waist (keep knees locked and chin tucked) until you feel a good stretch or discomfort in either the neck, mid, or lower back.

Breathe in three seconds then out three seconds—Fire Path Breathing

As you breathe in, you will rise a little; and then as you breathe out, you should bend more or sink down more at the waist. Don't push this too hard; let yourself sink down naturally.

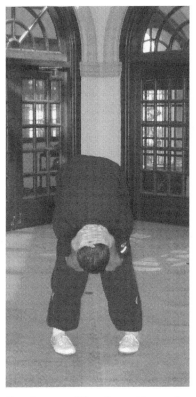
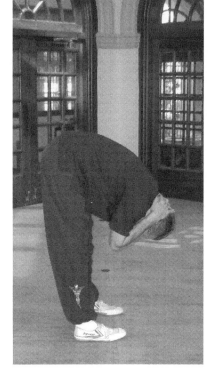

Beginner: Five breath cycles
Intermediate: Ten breath cycles
Advanced: Fifteen breath cycles

Key points

- Do not forget the visualization with the breathing.
- Keep the knees locked back and the chin tucked throughout the exercise.

- If holding the hands behind the neck or head puts to much pressure on the neck, then let your hands dangle in front of you.
- Do not overbend at the waist initially; just let your body sink down until the back or neck feels tight. That will be the starting position for this exercise.

Physical and Physiological Benefits

1. Increases cellular metabolic rate
2. Superoxygenates the blood
3. Continues to strengthen the diaphragm, improving breathing efficiency
4. Continues massage of internal organs
5. Continues improved oxygen and energy delivered to the brain
6. Continues the stimulation of the brain and brain activity
7. Continues the second heart's (the abdomen) ability to improve blood flow
8. Further charges the abdomen battery
9. Continues the release of endorphins that reduce pain and improve mood
10. Maximizes improvement in midline flexibility: Achilles tendons; calf muscles; hamstrings; lower, mid, and upper back; neck; and shoulders
11. Improves the energy meridians' movement of energy throughout the body

Potential Medical Health Benefits

1. Blood pressure
2. Resting heart rate
3. Asthma

4. Bowel function: constipation
5. Energy: chronic fatigue
6. Mood: depression and anxiety
7. Focus and attention
8. Memory
9. Lower and midback arthritis
10. Lower and midback chronic pain
11. Neck pain and arthritis
12. Chronic pain in general

Exercise No. 4 Dragon Swings Its Whiskers

- Position feet shoulder width apart.
- Bend the knees slightly.
- Hands start on the left side—left hand on the kidney and right on the chest.
- Rotate the spine from left to right so that both hands and arms swing out—right first then the left—in a big circle at chest level.

Right hand should stop by hitting/tapping the kidney area in the back, and left hand should stop by hitting/tapping the right chest area.

Then twist the spine the opposite way from right to left, letting the arms and hands swing out, with the left hand hitting the kidney area and the right hand hitting the chest at the end.

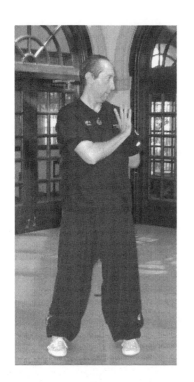
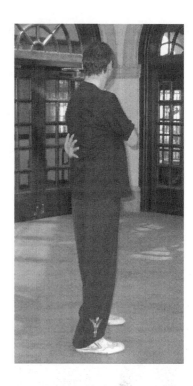
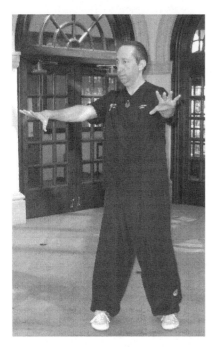
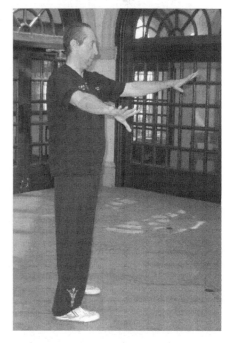

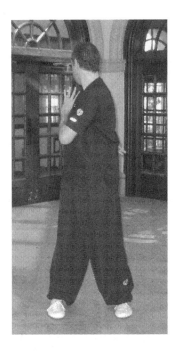 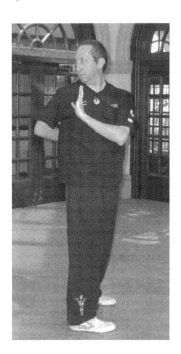

Beginner: Twenty-five times
Intermediate: Fifty times
Advanced: One hundred times

Key Points

- As you rotate, pick a spot behind you to look each time.
- Twisting your spine begins the rotation, not moving your arms.
- Swing your arms out as you twist with enough force to feel blood moving to your fingertips.
- As your arms swing out, *grab* the energy and pull it into your chest and kidneys when you tap them.

Physical and Physiological Benefits

1. Improves the energy meridians' movement of energy throughout the body

2. Continues the massage of the internal organs, stimulating and energizing them
3. Continues the release of endorphins that reduce pain and improve mood
4. Maximizes spinal flexibility
5. Improves hip and pelvic muscle strength and endurance
6. Brings energy to the lungs, kidneys, and adrenal glands
7. Brings blood to the fingertips
8. Improves balance and coordination

Potential Medical Health Benefits

1. Asthma
2. Bowel function
3. Energy
4. Lower and midback pain and arthritis
5. Hand and finger pain and arthritis
6. Chronic pain in general
7. Balance, preventing falls
8. Continues to improve mood

Fire Element:

Improving Cardiovascular Performance and Energy

Exercise No. 5 Stand High to Embrace the Moon

- Position feet more than shoulder width apart.
- Turn both feet slightly outward.
- Squat down with your back straight as low as you can, hands to your sides.
- Push up from your heels with your legs to a standing position.

- Bring arms up out along your sides and over your head, clapping them together over your head.
- Sink back down as low as you can, bringing the arms back to your sides.

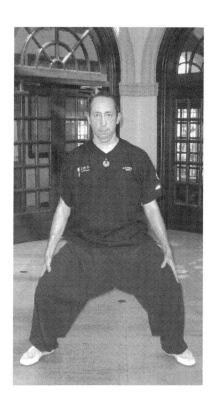 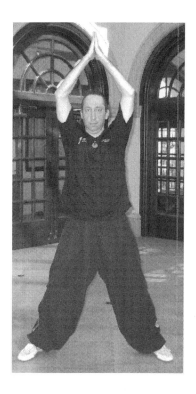

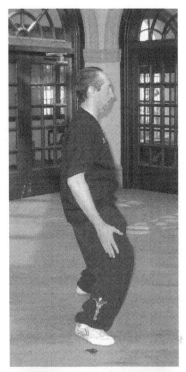

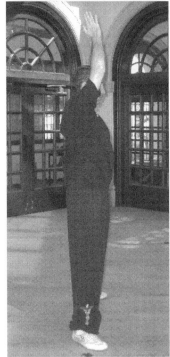

Beginner: Twenty-five times
Intermediate: Fifty times
Advanced: One hundred times

Key Points

- Keep the back as straight as you can. Do not hunch over; this will minimize the tension on the knees.
- Do this as quickly as you can, but be careful you don't lose your balance.
- Clapping your hands together over your head rotates your shoulder, giving you a better upper body stretch and exercises the shoulder more completely.
- Clapping also stimulates the nerve endings in the hand and fingers.
- Sink down as low as you can. Push yourself.

Physical and Physiological Benefits

1. Further increases cellular metabolic rate for maximal calorie burn
2. Improves thigh, hip, pelvic, lower back, and gluteus strength and endurance
3. Improves shoulder and chest strength, stamina, and flexibility
4. Stimulates the nerve endings in the hands and fingers
5. Increases thigh, hip, pelvic, and lower back bone marrow health and bone density
6. Continues maximal oxygen and energy delivered to the brain
7. Continues the stimulation of the brain and brain activity
8. Begins to activate the third heart to improve blood flow (the calf muscles)
9. Continues the release of endorphins that reduce pain and improve mood
10. Continues to stimulate the energy meridians

11. Improves cardiovascular performance
12. Improves balance and coordination

Potential Medical Health Benefits
1. Blood pressure reduction
2. Heart rate reduction
3. Blood sugar consumption: diabetes
4. Increase in good HDL cholesterol that helps eliminate plaque in your arteries
5. Asthma
6. Strengthens the blood by reducing internal inflammatory factors that accelerate aging
7. Arthritis of the knees-hips-lumbar-shoulders-hands-fingers, and improves
8. Energy
9. Mood
10. Focus and memory
11. Balance, preventing falls

Exercise No. 6 Throw the Ball

- Position feet shoulder width apart.
- Extend the arms and hands forward in front of you, lifting them to shoulder height.
- Lock out the elbows but keep the shoulders relaxed.
- Cup the thumb *over* the other four fingers (index to pinkie).

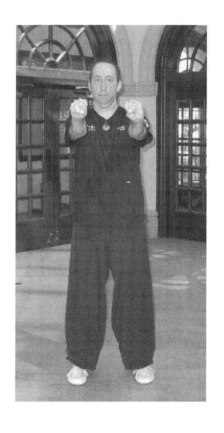
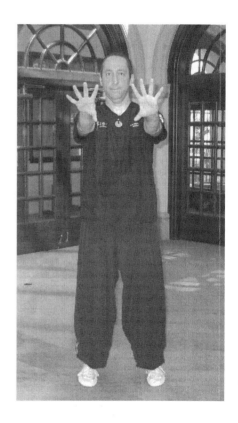

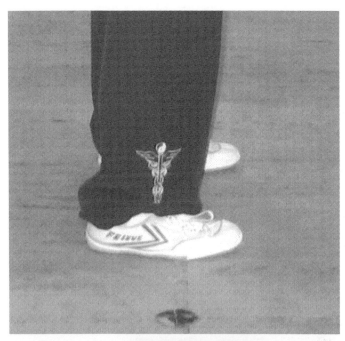

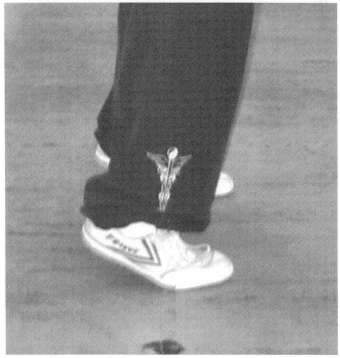

Flick your fingers off of the thumbs like you're flicking water off them. At the same time, push up off your heels and onto your toes and then drop back down onto your heels.

Do this as fast as you can.

Beginner: Fifty times
Intermediate: One hundred times
Advanced: Two hundred times

Key Points:

- Flick and push up at the same time and repeat this as fast as you can but keep those elbow locked. It's harder than you may think.
- Drop back down onto your heels so that you feel your body shake a little—not too hard so you hurt yourself.
- Try and keep your shoulders relaxed as you do this exercise.

Physical and Physiological Benefits

1. Further increases cellular metabolic rate for maximal calorie burn
2. Improves lower leg, hand, arm, shoulder, and chest strength and endurance
3. Provides oxygen to the fingertips and toes
4. Stimulates the nerve endings of the fingers and toes
5. Continues maximal oxygen and energy delivered to the brain
6. Continues the stimulation of the brain and brain activity
7. Improves the activity of the third heart to improve blood flow (the calf muscles)
8. Continues the release of endorphins that reduce pain and improve mood

9. Continues to stimulate energy flow through the meridians
10. Improves cardiovascular performance
11. Improves balance and coordination
12. Improves leg, hip, and pelvic strength and endurance

Potential Medical Health Benefits

1. Blood pressure
2. Heart rate
3. Blood sugar consumption: diabetes
4. Increase in good HDL cholesterol that helps eliminate plaque in your arteries
5. Asthma
6. Strengthens the blood by reducing inflammatory factors
7. Arthritis of the lower back, toes, feet, ankles, shoulders, hands, and fingers
8. Energy
9. Mood, focus, and memory
10. Balance, preventing falls

Earth Element:

Improving Core Strength, Stamina, and Balance

Exercise No. 7 Taoist Horse Stance

- Position feet shoulder width apart.
- Turn toes in forty-five-degree angle.
- Bend the knees and squat down as low as you feel comfortable. Don't let the knees touch. *It is OK to start high.*
- Lift head and look straight up, arching the back, and then look forward, keeping that back arched or as straight as possible.

- Lift arm and hand up in front and point the fingers first straight up then twist them so they are pointing toward each other. Keep the arms out when you do this.
- Now place the right hand on top of the left so the right thumb is on top of the left pinkie.

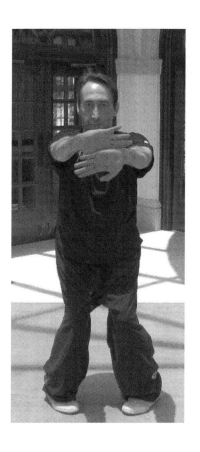
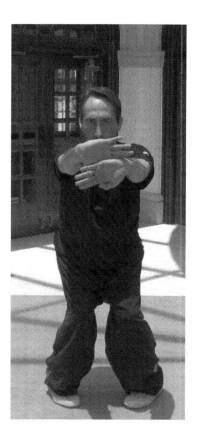

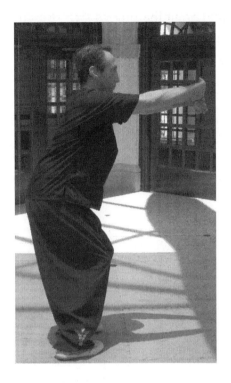 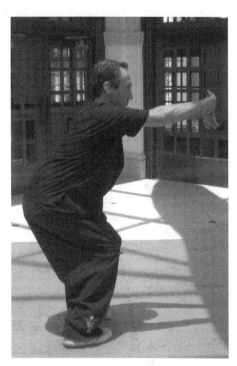

Take a deep breathe for three seconds.
Exhale three seconds and sink down on your legs and push out with your hands.
This is one cycle.

Relax and breathe in, rising a little but keeping the arms locked out.
Breathe out and sink further, pushing out with the hands.

Beginner: Five breath cycles
Intermediate: Ten breaths
Advanced: Fifteen breaths

Key Points

- Initially, take your time getting into this position and adjust your position to eliminate any discomfort you may feel.

- Relax the arms and legs as you exhale but keep the arms locked out. Tighten the legs as you sink and the arms as you push out with the hands. Keep the hands in the proper position with the right on top of the left.
- If there is too much pressure on the lower back or if it hurts, lean forward until that goes away.
- Start high initially but then start at a lower position as you gain in strength. Push yourself!
- You do not have to sink down on the legs much as you exhale to make this effective.

Physical and Physiological Benefits

1. Further increases cellular metabolic rate for maximal calorie burn
2. Improves thigh, hip, pelvic, lower back, abdominal, and gluteus strength and endurance
3. Improves shoulder, chest, and arm strength and endurance
4. Increases thigh, hip, pelvic, lower back, arm, and shoulder bone and bone marrow health
5. Continues maximal oxygen and energy delivered to the brain
6. Continues the stimulation of the brain and brain activity
7. Supports the immune system by stimulating the bone marrow
8. Continues the release of endorphins that reduce pain and improve mood
9. Continues to stimulate energy flow through the meridians
10. Improves balance and coordination

Potential Medical Health Benefits

1. Improvement in blood pressure and reduction in heart rate
2. Blood sugar consumption: diabetes
3. Increase in good HDL cholesterol that helps eliminate plaque in your arteries
4. Improvement in asthma

5. Reduction of internal inflammatory factors that age us
6. Improvement in immune function
7. Improvement in bone density: Prevents and improves osteopenia and osteoporosis
8. Improvement in arthritis of the toes, feet, ankles, shoulders, hands, and fingers
9. Improvement in balance, preventing falls
10. Improvement in energy, mood, focus, and memory.

Exercise No. 8 Tai Chi Mountain Climbing Stance

- Position feet shoulder width apart.
- Pull left leg back and turn the foot forty-five degrees outward and lock the knee.
- Move right leg forward and bend the right knee as low as you can go—do not let your knee go past your toes.

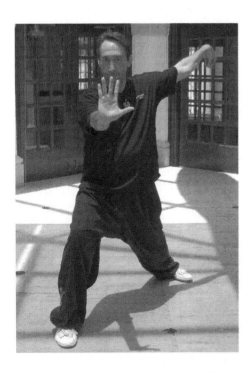
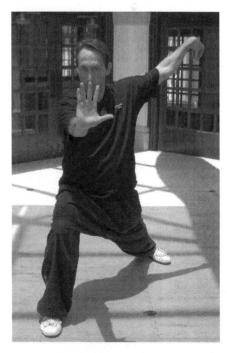

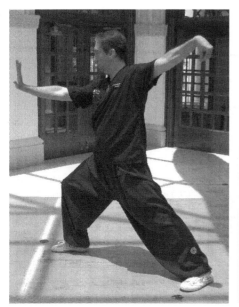 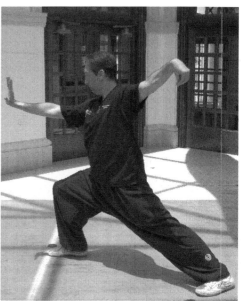

It is OK to start in a high.

Extend right arm directly in front, shoulder height, in the same direction as the front leg and pull back the hand and fingers toward you, then push the middle finger *out away from you*. *This is called the Tai Chi Palm.* Bring the left arm up with hand at the level of your left ear, lock the elbow out, move the hand and arm back, and point the hand down like your are dropping sand onto your left foot. Your hand should be *over* your left foot. You should feel a stretch across your left chest and shoulder. If it is painful, then shift your arm more forward.

Take a deep breathe for three seconds.
Exhale three seconds and sink down on your right leg. Push out *with your right hand and* down *with your left hand.*

This is one cycle.

Relax and breathe in, rising a little but keeping the arms locked out.
Breathe out and sink further, pushing out with right and down with left.

Beginner: Five breath cycles
Intermediate: Ten breaths
Advanced: Fifteen breaths

Switch and repeat on the opposite side.

Key points

- Pull the wrist and fingers back as best you can and push the middle finger forward.
- The hand that is back should be at ear level, with elbow locked out, and hand pointed down over the foot like you were sprinkling sand on it.
- Keep the knee of the back leg locked.
- Feet should be at least a shoulder width apart.
- Start at a lower position as you gain in strength.
- Try and turn your hips more forward with time and you gain in flexibility. This maximizes groin and hip stretch.

Physical and Physiological Benefits

1. Further increases cellular metabolic rate for maximal calorie burn
2. Improves thigh, hip, pelvic, lower back, abdominal, and gluteus strength, endurance, and flexibility
3. Improves shoulder, chest, and arm strength, endurance, and flexibility
4. Increases thigh, hip, pelvic, lower back, arm, and shoulder bone and bone marrow health
5. Continues maximal oxygen and energy delivered to the brain
6. Continues the stimulation of the brain and brain activity
7. Continues the release of endorphins that reduce pain and improve mood
8. Continues to stimulate energy flow through the meridians

9. Activates the energy meridians to improve energy throughout the body
10. Improves balance and coordination

Potential Medical Health Benefits

1. Improvement in blood pressure and reduction in heart rate
2. Blood sugar consumption: diabetes
3. Increase in good HDL cholesterol that helps eliminate plaque in your arteries
4. Asthma
5. Reduction of internal inflammatory factors
6. Immune function
7. Improvement in bone density: prevents and improves osteopenia and osteoporosis
8. Improvement in balance and prevents falls
9. Energy, mood, focus, and memory

Water Element:

Maximizing Bone Hardness and Immunity

Exercise No. 9 Pushing the Millstone

- Position feet shoulder width apart.
- Move left foot back and turn out to forty-five degrees.
- Move right foot forward with toe pointed forward, sink down and widen the stance to get as low as possible but stay comfortable.
- Your weight at the start should be about 50/50 front and back leg.

Stretch your fingers out with both hands and then put them together so that the index finger and thumb of each hand touch, making a diamond. Place the diamond at waist level and parallel to the ground, starting over the right knee.

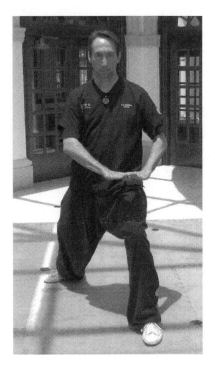
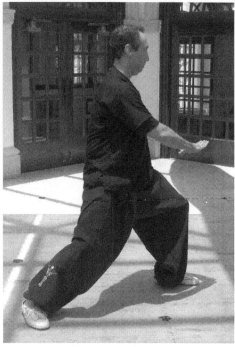

Breathe in and at the same time twist right at the waist. Bring the hands in toward your abdomen, turn them across your abdomen and over the right hip as we twist, and push back on your front foot, shifting most of the weight to the back foot.

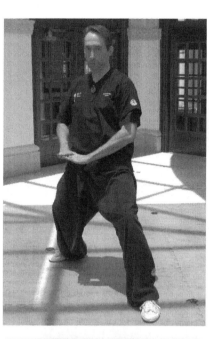
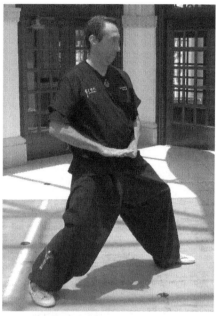
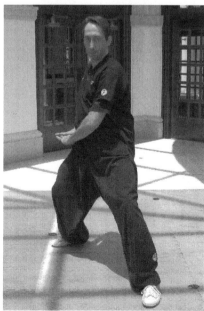
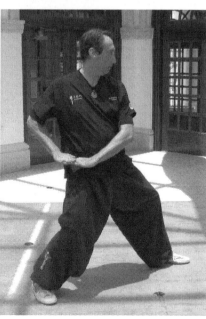

Breathe out and push the hands out and twist left. Push off the back foot, transferring the weight more to your front foot and bring your hands back over your knee. **This completes *one breath cycle.***

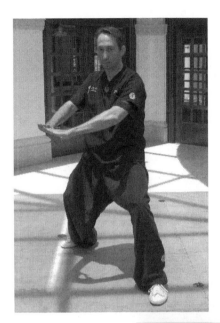
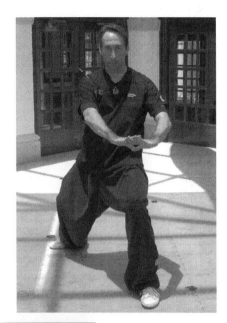
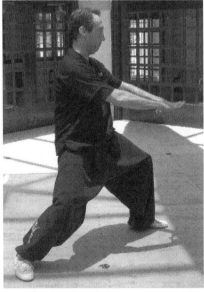

Breathe in for three seconds and out for four seconds.

Switch and repeat on the opposite side.

Beginner: Three breath cycles
Intermediate: Six breaths
Advanced: Nine breaths

Key Points

- Keep the hands together, forming the diamond, and keep the diamond parallel to the ground at all times.
- When shifting your weight, you do not have to move much.
- When you shift your weight from front to back to front, try not to bob your head up. Keep your head at one level, this will take time.
- Do not rush through this exercise; this exercise is *key* in sealing in all the energy you created to use later on in the day.

Physical and Physiological Benefits

1. Further increases cellular metabolic rate for maximal calorie burn
2. Improves thigh, hip, pelvic, lower back, abdominal, and gluteus strength and endurance
3. Improves shoulder, chest, and arm strength and endurance
4. Increases thigh, hip, pelvic, lower back, arm, and shoulder bone and bone marrow health
5. Continues maximal oxygen and energy delivered to the brain
6. Continues the stimulation of the brain and brain activity
7. Continues the release of endorphins that reduce pain and improve mood
8. Continues to stimulate energy flow through the meridians
9. Improves balance and coordination

Potential Medical Health Benefits

1. Improvement in blood pressure and reduction in heart rate
2. Blood sugar consumption: diabetes
3. Increase in good HDL cholesterol that helps eliminate plaque in your arteries
4. Asthma
5. Reduction of internal inflammatory factors
6. Maximizes immune function
7. Maximizes improvement in bone density: prevents and improves osteopenia and osteoporosis
8. Maximizes improvement in balance and coordination to prevents falls
9. Energy, mood, focus, and memory

Recapping

1. **Most importantly, have fun.**
2. **Give yourself the first week to get familiar with the exercises of the program.**
3. **If any of the exercises are uncomfortable, adjust your positioning until that discomfort is resolved.**
4. **These excesses are targeted to supercharge your metabolic rate on *all* levels so you can rip through calories and accelerate your weight loss and then keep it off.**
5. **This exercise program is not just about weight; it's about improving your health and fitness as well, so everyone can incorporate it as part of their morning routine.**

One Final Note

I frequently ask my patients the following question:

"What are you working so hard for?"

They look back at me, puzzled.

I continue, "Unless you exercise and begin to take care of yourself, it seems to me that you're working very hard every day to be *disabled*! Which color wheelchair do you want me to order?"

People work very hard their whole life just to become permanently disabled . . . I see this every day.

Let's change this by making a promise to ourselves starting right *now*.

About the Author

Michael Keller, MD, is a family practice physician and part owner of Southwest Family Practice, which currently has four clinic sites in the Phoenix metropolitan area. He also is on the Zen Wellness Instructor Certification Board of Directors and is the medical director of the Zen Wellness—Avondale, Arizona, location.

Dr. Keller is a second-degree black belt instructor registered with the United Martial Arts Association of America with proficiencies in the following forms—Tiger and Crane, Northern Chinese Long Fist, and Tai Chi—and is a certified first degree Doh Yi master with the International Doh Yi Federation and is a certified Chi Fit Medical Chi Gong (Qigong) instructor through Zen Wellness and the National Qigong Association.

Dr. Keller was born in the small farming community of Moline, Illinois, in 1967, where he graduated top 5 percent of his class in high school in 1985. He then received his bachelors of science degree in biochemistry in 1989 through the University of Illinois at Urbana—Champaign. Dr. Keller was then accepted into the University of Illinois at Chicago College of Medicine Medical Program, where he received his doctor of medicine in 1994. Following graduation, he was accepted into Resurrection Family Practice Residency program through Resurrection Hospital in North Chicago where he successfully accomplished his American Academy of Family Practice specialty training. Dr. Keller is currently board certified in family practice and has active diplomat status.

Dr. Keller has been involved with medical and general scientific research since his undergraduate training with scholarships awarded for research through the American Heart Association and both the Department of Physiology and Department of Hematology and Oncology at the University Illinois at Chicago. Dr. Keller has publications in critical medical and scientific journals such as *Circulation Research, Biophysical Journal, Proceedings of the National Academy of Sciences*, the *Regulation of Hemoglobin Switching,* and *Blood*.

In 2001, Dr. Keller created and published a free comprehensive health care magazine called *Health Focus*, which was distributed throughout the Phoenix metropolitan area. Thirty thousand copies were distributed at the launch. The magazine was developed to provide relevant medical information that included all specialty fields, locations, and information relating to all of the area hospitals, up-to-date information on cutting-edge medications, and included current relative, local, and national government political information as well as access to local and state representatives, congressmen, and senators. The magazine was a success from its launch.

Dr. Keller is continuing his medical research with Zen Wellness where he assisted in setting up Zen Illuminations, a cutting-edge biological age testing and tracking program. This program uses state-of-the-art Polar Body Age Testing equipment (as used by Dr. Oz on *Oprah* and in all of the Lifetime Fitness gyms across the country) to establish the differences between actual physical body age to actual chronological body age in years and then tracks the tremendous effect that Zen Wellness and United Martial Arts Training has on significantly reversing the aging process.

Dr. Keller discovered the medical benefits of martial arts, especially Chi Gong, Zen Yoga, and Tai Chi when he found himself struggling with his own health. In 2005, Dr. Keller was taking medications for diabetes, high cholesterol, high blood pressure, and peaked to a robust 265 pounds in weight. He was suffering from stress, was tired all the time, cranky (according to his children); and his relationships with his family were suffering. In the past four years that he has been involved with Eastern medical philosophical disciplines, he has dropped sixty pounds in weight, is no longer a diabetic, no longer suffers from high blood pressure, has more energy, has a very low heart rate, is no longer a victim of stress, and most importantly enjoys a more interactive and positive relationship with his family. Dr. Keller is slowly incorporating more of the Eastern ideals into his medical practice and finds that a balance of classic Western medicine and the benefits of Chi Gong, Zen Yoga, and Tai Chi have provided the most impressive results in curing medical problems within his practice.

Dr. Keller is currently hard in training for his third-degree black belt, which he hopes to accomplish no later than 2010. He is also assisting in Tai Chi instruction within the Zen Wellness community in the Phoenix metropolitan area.

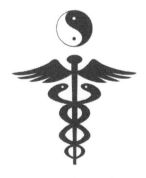

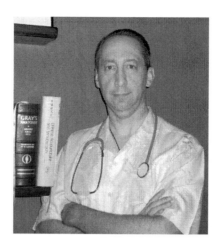

Michael R. Keller, MD

You can find me at www.medicalzen.com. Come take a look.

Dr. Michael Keller strongly encourages all individuals to involve their physician in the management of any chronic medical conditions. Medical Zen: Fit in 15 should not be used as a substitute for appropriate medical care or in lieu of recommended or prescribed medical treatments. Daily routine exercise is part of a healthy way of life.

would like to thank the following:

Master Michael Leone who can be found at www.ZenWellness.com, www.AZKungFu.com, www.ZenYoga.com

Master Jason Campbell who can be found at www.ZenWellness.com, www.AZKungFu.com, www.ZenYoga.com, www.zenbusinessbootcamp.com

Colleen Inman who can be found at www.cinman.me

Michael J. Swanzk who can be found at www.martialgolf.net

Index

Metal Element: 13
  Exercise No. 1
  Embrace the Heart, 14

  Exercise No. 2
  Gather the Sun
  and Press the Earth, 18

Wood Element: 25
  Exercise No. 3
  Midline Stretch, 25

  Exercise No. 4
  Dragon Swings Its Whiskers, 28

Fire Element: 31
  Exercise No. 5
  Stand High to
  Embrace the Moon, 31

  Exercise No. 6
  Throw the Ball, 35

Earth Element: 39
  Exercise No. 7
  Taoist Horse Stance, 39

  Exercise No. 8
  Tai Chi
  Mountain Climbing Stance, 43

Water Element: 46
  Exercise No. 9
  Pushing the Millstone, 46

Made in the USA
Lexington, KY
17 April 2011